Staying Healthy

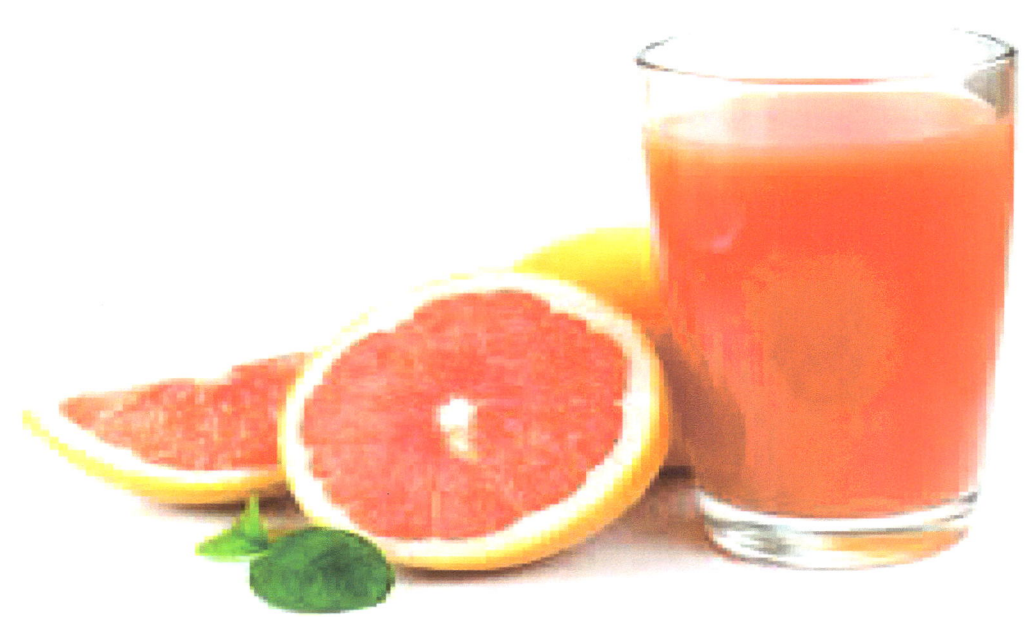

STAYING HEALTH

Library of Congress Cataloging- in Publication Data

ISBN: 1514268116

www.LULU.COM

Printed in U.S.A.

Contents

Introduction

The thirst quenching juices on the market can be expensive. The quest for finding the most nutritional juice for your specific needs can be exhausting.

My journey to find inexpensive and nutritional juices brought me to this journey. I have put together this book to share with anyone who has the same desires. I hope you enjoy yourself!!

2
Juicing Recipes

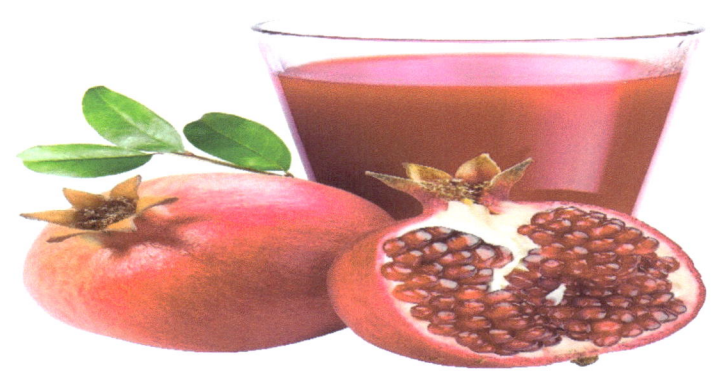

Green Bouquet

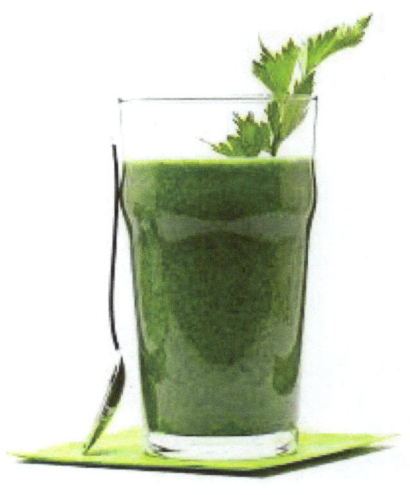

¼ cup of bananas sliced

½ cup of kale chopped

½ cup of sliced apple

¼ cup of blueberries

1 tsp of fresh mint chopped

3 tbsp of honey

Place washed Kale in blender or nutri- bullet first then place remaining fruits in the blender or nutria bullet and add half of cup of water and pour in honey. Blend for 2 minutes then pour over ice.

A Raspberry Beet

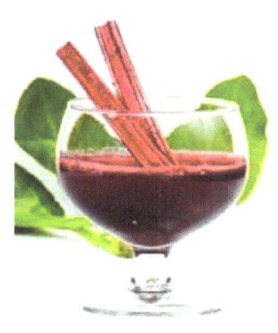

¼ cup of beets sliced

¼ cup of raspberries

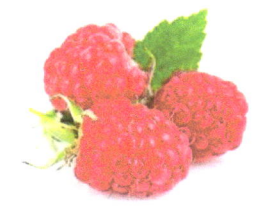

½ cup of kale

½ tbsp of fresh mint chopped

2 tbsp of fresh squeeze lemon juice

3 tbsp of honey

Place washed kale in nutri bullet or blender then place remaining fruits in the blender or nutria bullet and half of cup of water and pour honey. Blend for 2 minutes then pour over ice.

ALOE VERA DELIGHT

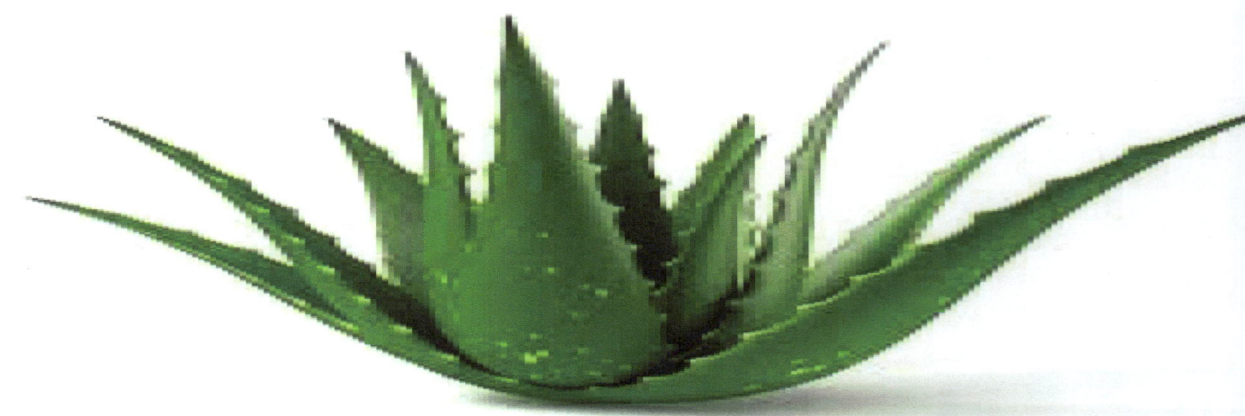

3 tbsp of aloe vera with skin off

2 tsp of fresh squeeze lemon juice

½ cup of kale

½ cup of sliced strawberries

¼ cup of blackberries

4 tbsp of honey

Cut skin off of aloe vera and place it in blender. Place washed kale in nutri bullet or blender then place remaining fruits in the blender or nutria bullet and half of cup of water and pour honey. Blend for 2 minutes then pour over ice.

Strawberry Twist

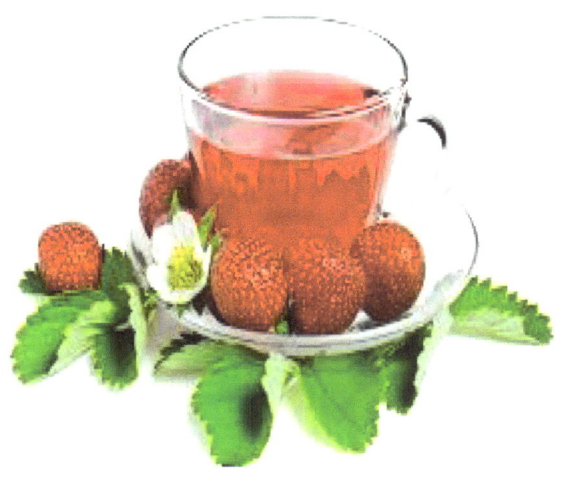

½ cup of sliced strawberries

¼ cup of blackberries

¼ cup of blueberries

½ cup of kale

¼ cup of collard greens

2 tsp of fresh squeeze lemon juice

4 tbsp of honey

Place washed kale in nutri bullet or blender then place remaining fruits in the blender or nutria bullet and half of cup of water and pour honey. Blend for 2 minutes then pour over ice.

Sweet Potatoe Variety

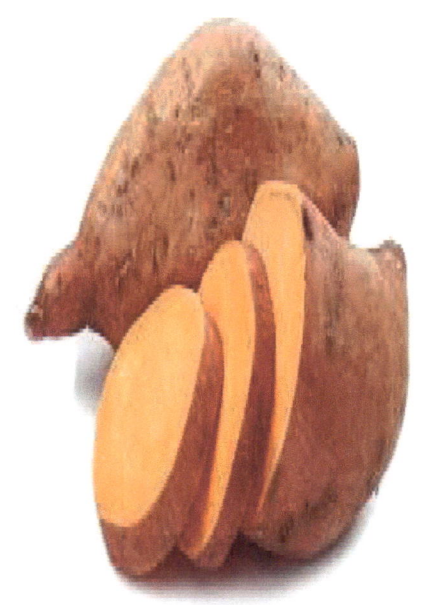

½ cup of sliced sweet potatoes

¼ cup of sliced strawberries

¼ cup of blueberries

½ cup of kale

2 tsp of fresh squeeze lime juice

4 tbsp of honey

Cut skin off of sweet potatoes and slice and wash. Place washed kale in nutri bullet or blender then place remaining fruits in the blender or nutria bullet and half of cup of water and pour honey. Blend for 2 minutes then pour over ice.

Red Apple

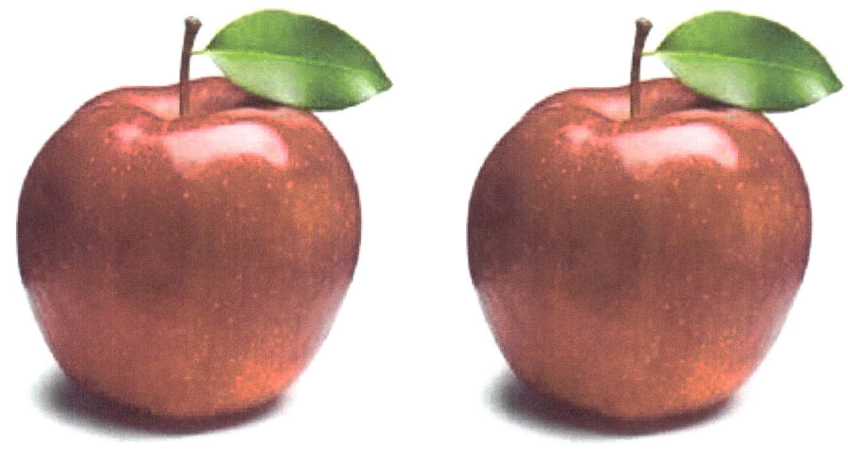

1 apple

¼ cup of water

¼ cup of strawberries

¼ cup of raspberries

4 tbsp of honey

Place sliced apples skin off and water remaining fruit and honey in blender or nutri bullet. Blend for 1 minute serve over ice.

Red Cabbage

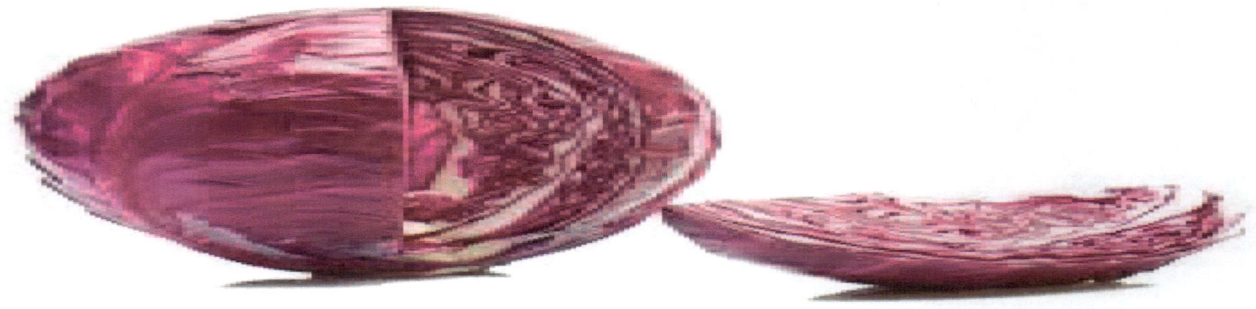

½ cup of chopped red cabbage

¼ cup of black berries

¼ cup of strawberries

½ cup of kale

½ cup of pineapples

5 tbsp of honey

½ cup of water

Cut red cabbage into strips and wash. Place washed kale in nutri bullet or blender then place remaining fruits in the blender or nutria bullet and half of cup of water and pour honey. Blend for 2 minutes then pour over ice.

Piercing Pears

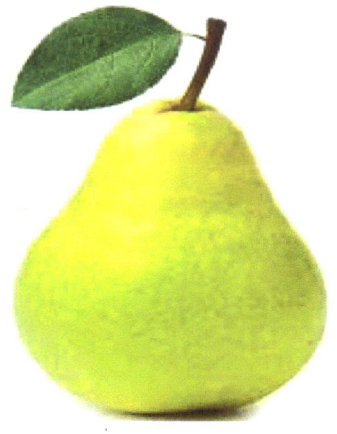

½ cup of chopped pears skin removed

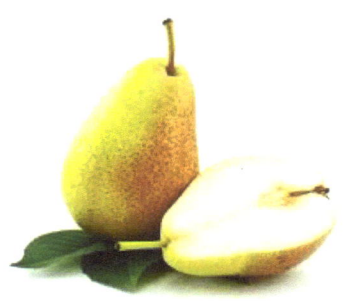

1/4 cup of oranges

½ cup of kale

¼ cup of pineapples

2 tbsp of grapefruit juice

4 tbsp of honey

Cut pears remove skin. Place washed kale in nutri bullet or blender then place remaining fruits in the blender or nutria bullet and half of cup of water and pour honey. Blend for 2 minutes then pour over ice.

Celebrating Celery

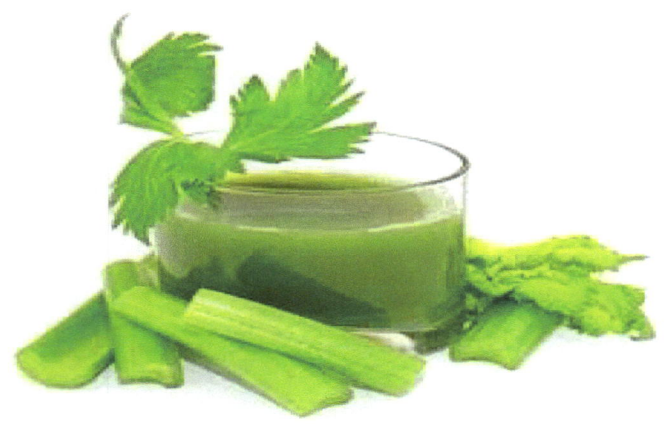

½ cup of chopped celery

½ cup of kale

1 tbsp of fresh squeeze lime juice

½ cup of blackberries

¼ cup of blueberries

½ cup of water

5 tbsp of honey

Cut celery and rinse. Place washed kale in nutri bullet or blender then place remaining fruits in the blender or nutria bullet and half of cup of water and pour honey. Blend for 2 minutes then pour over ice.

Ginger Kick

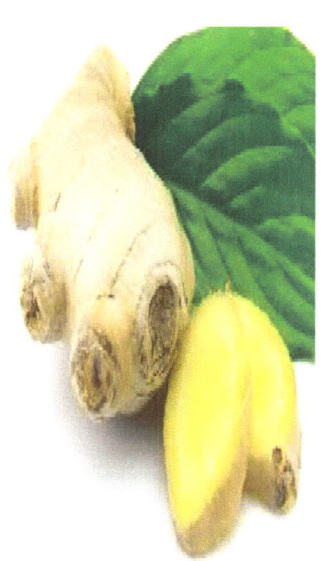

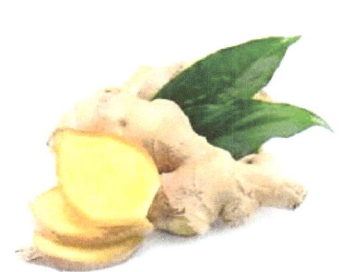

3 small strips skin remove ginger root

½ cup of kale

½ cup of strawberries

½ cup of pears

½ cup of water

5 tbsp of honey

Cut ginger root and remove skin from pears. Place washed kale in nutri bullet or blender then place remaining fruits in the blender or nutria bullet and half of cup of water and pour honey. Blend for 2 minutes then pour over ice.

Tasty Grapefruit

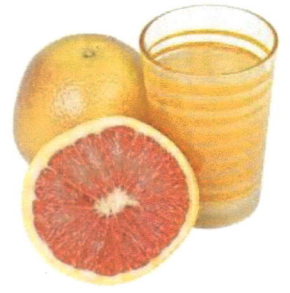 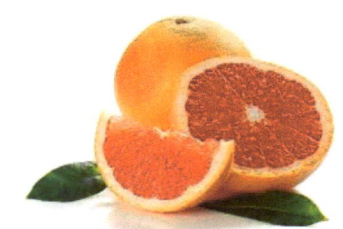 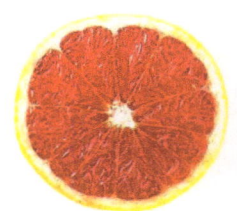 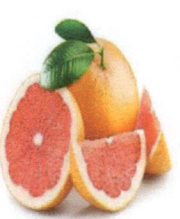

½ cup of grapefruit skin removed

½ cup of fresh orange juice

½ cup of pears skin removed

½ cup of blueberries

½ cup of raspberries

½ cup of water

6 tbsp of honey

Cut grapefruit and remove skin. Place washed kale in nutri bullet or blender then place remaining fruits in the blender or nutria bullet and half of cup of water and pour honey. Blend for 2 minutes then pour over ice.

Preppy Pineapple

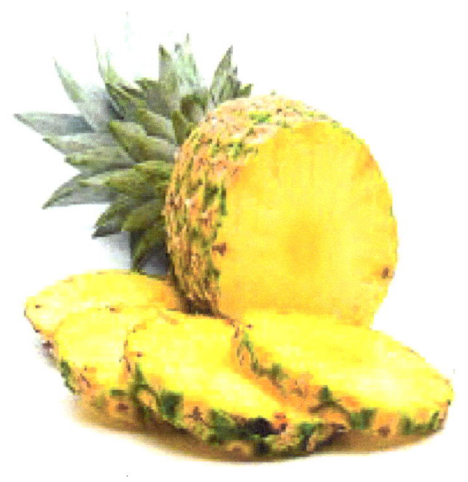

1/2 cup of pineapple

½ cup of kale

½ cup of blueberries

¼ cup of pomegranate

½ cup of strawberries

½ cup of water

4tbsp of honey

Cut pineapple skin removed and skin removed from pears. Place washed kale in nutri bullet or blender then place remaining fruits in the blender or nutria bullet and half of cup of water and pour honey. Blend for 2 minutes then pour over ice.

Slushy Pomegranate

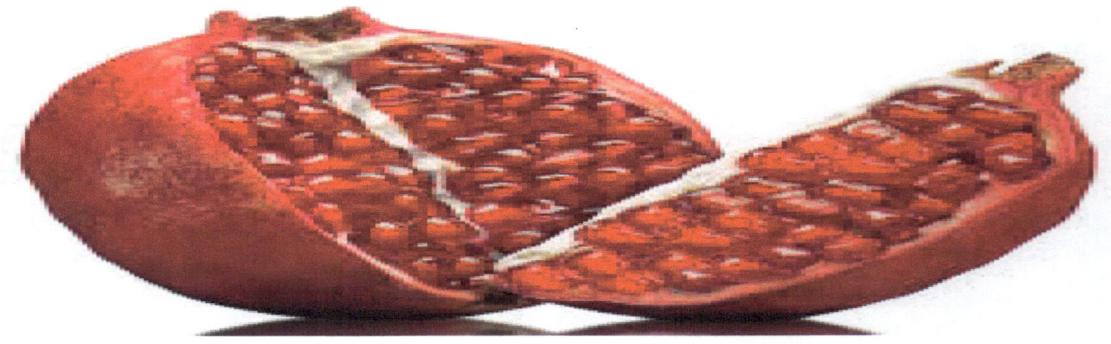

½ cup of pomegranate seeds

½ cup of kale

½ cup of raspberries

½ cup of strawberries

½ cup of grapes

4 ice cubes

½ cup of water

5tbsp of honey

Place washed kale in nutri bullet or blender then place remaining fruits in the blender or nutria bullet and half of cup of water and pour honey. Blend for 2 minutes then pour over ice.

ONION

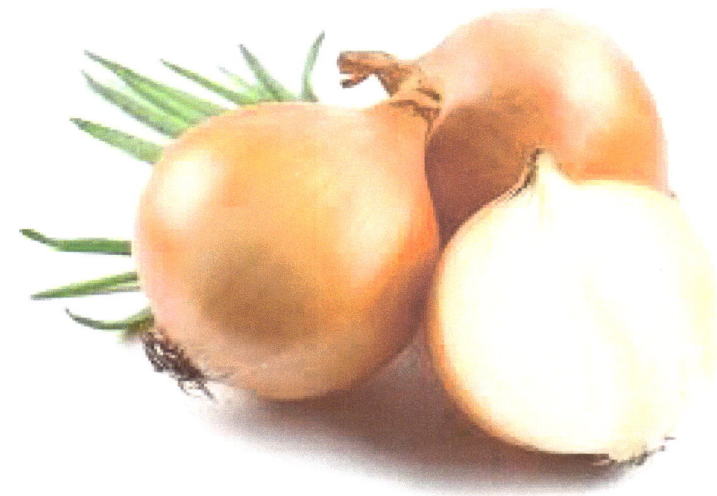

¼ cup of chopped onions

½ cup kale

½ cup of pineapple

½ cup of chopped pears skin removed

½ cup of blueberries

½ cup of strawberries

½ cup of water

6tbsp of honey

Cut onions remove skin and remove skin from pears. Place washed kale in nutri bullet or blender then place remaining fruits in the blender or nutria bullet and half of cup of water and pour honey. Blend for 2 minutes then pour over ice.

Bountiful Bananas

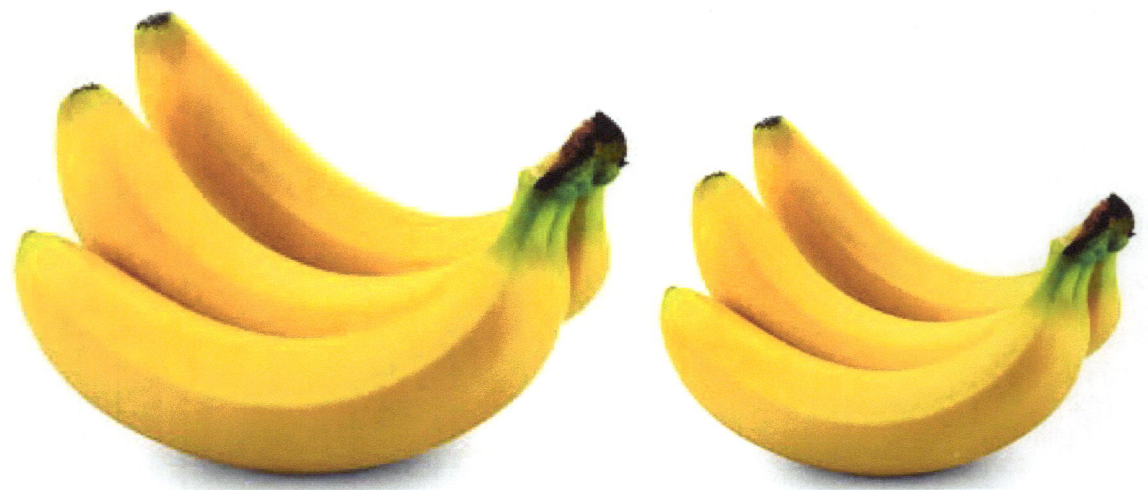

1 whole banana skin removed

½ cup of kale

½ cup of pineapples

½ cup of blackberries

¼ cup of blueberries

¼ cup of cherries

½ cup of water

4tbsp of honey

Slice banana remove skin and take seeds out of cherries remove skin from pineapples. Place washed kale in nutri bullet or blender then place remaining fruits in the blender or nutria bullet and half of cup of water and pour honey. Blend for 2 minutes then pour over ice.

O Orange

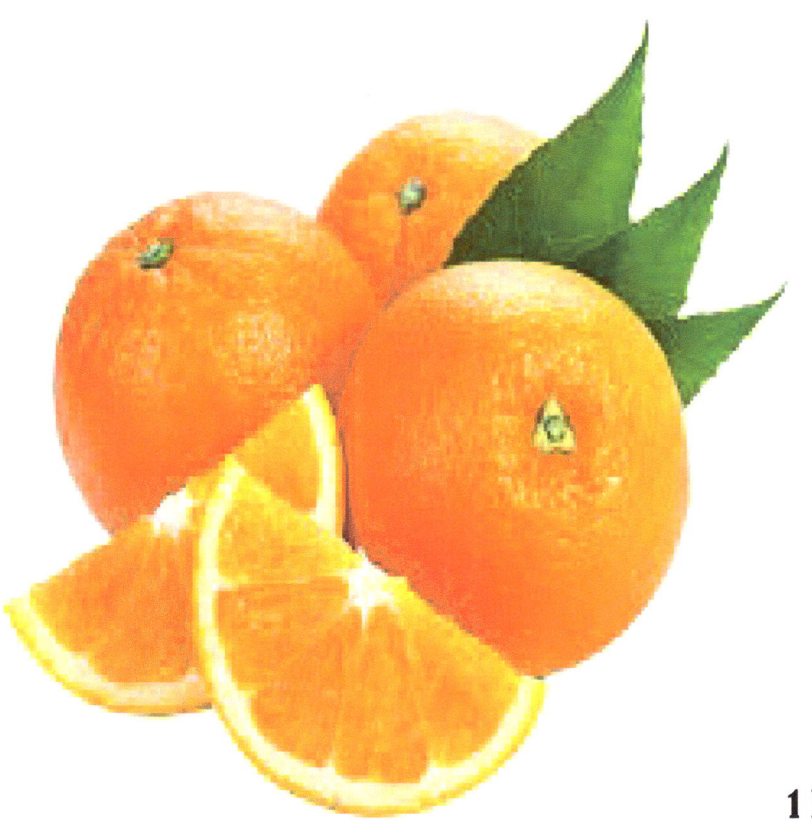

1 Large orange skin removed

½ cup of pineapple skin removed

½ cup of pomegranate seeds

¼ cup of kale

½ cup of water

3tbsp of honey

Remove skin from orange and remove skin from pineapple. Place washed kale in nutri bullet or blender then place remaining fruits in the blender or nutria bullet and half of cup of water and pour honey. Blend for 2 minutes then pour over ice.

Fresh Mint

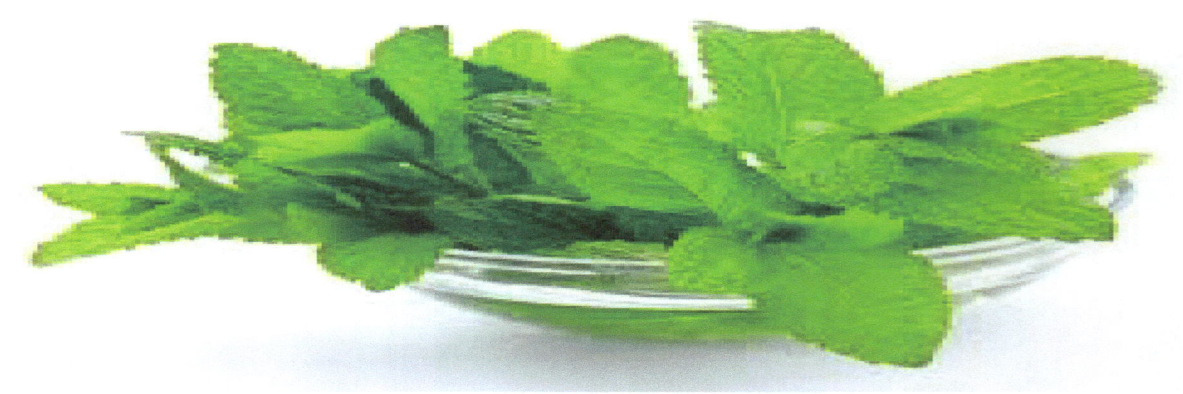

½ cup of fresh mint

½ cup of kale

½ cup of pineapple

½ cup of raspberries

½ cup of strawberries

½ cup of water

5tbsp of honey

Remove skin from pineapple. Place washed kale in nutri bullet or blender then place remaining fruits in the blender or nutria bullet and half of cup of water and pour honey. Blend for 2 minutes then pour over ice.

Can Can Cantaloupe

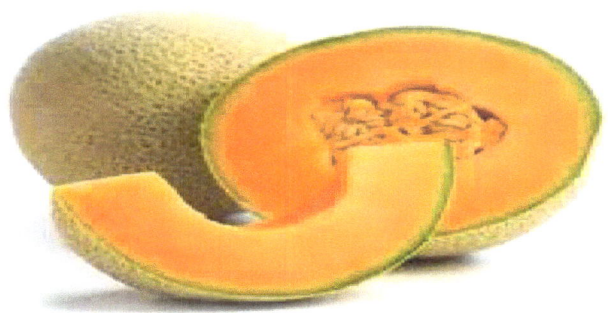

½ cup of cantaloupe skin removed

½ cup of kale

½ cup of pineapples

½ cup of orange skin removed

½ cup of blueberries

½ cup of blackberries

½ cup of water

4tbsp of honey

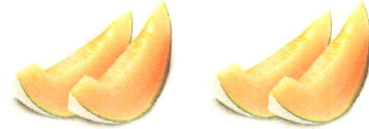

Place washed kale in nutri bullet or blender then place remaining fruits in the blender or nutria bullet and half of cup of water and pour honey. Blend for 2 minutes then pour over ice.

Lemon Lime

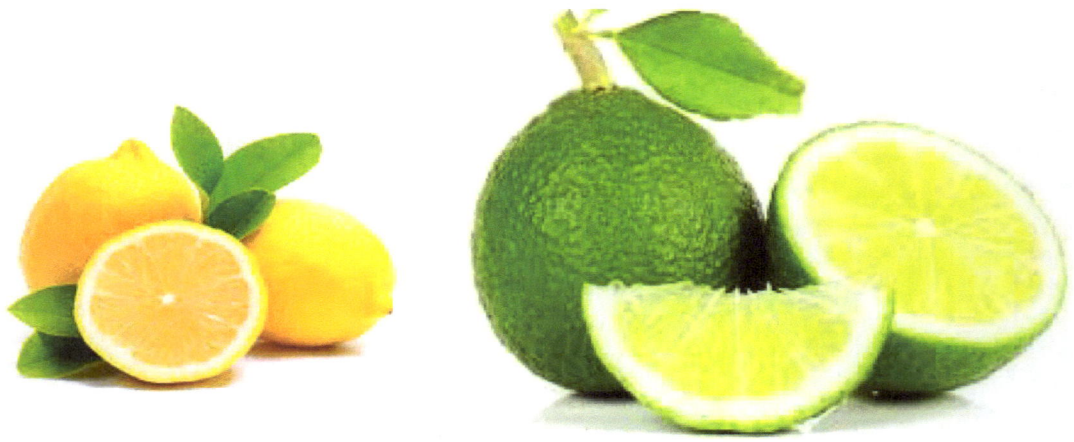

3tbsp of freshly squeeze lemon

3tbsp of freshly squeeze lime

½ cup of strawberries

½ cup of raspberries

½ cup of kale

½ cup of water

5tbsp of honey

Place washed kale in nutri bullet or blender then place remaining fruits in the blender or nutria bullet and half of cup of water and pour honey. Blend for 2 minutes then pour over ice.

Red Bell Pepper

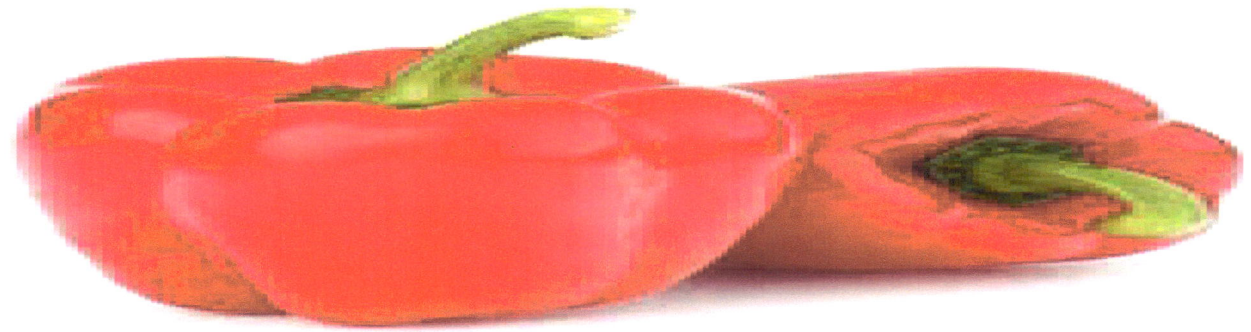

½ cup of chopped red bell pepper

½ cup of strawberries

½ cup of pears skin removed

½ cup of blueberries

½ cup of kale

5tbsp of honey

½ cup of water

Remove stem from bell pepper. Place washed kale in nutri bullet or blender then place remaining fruits in the blender or nutria bullet and half of cup of water and pour honey. Blend for 2 minutes then pour over ice.

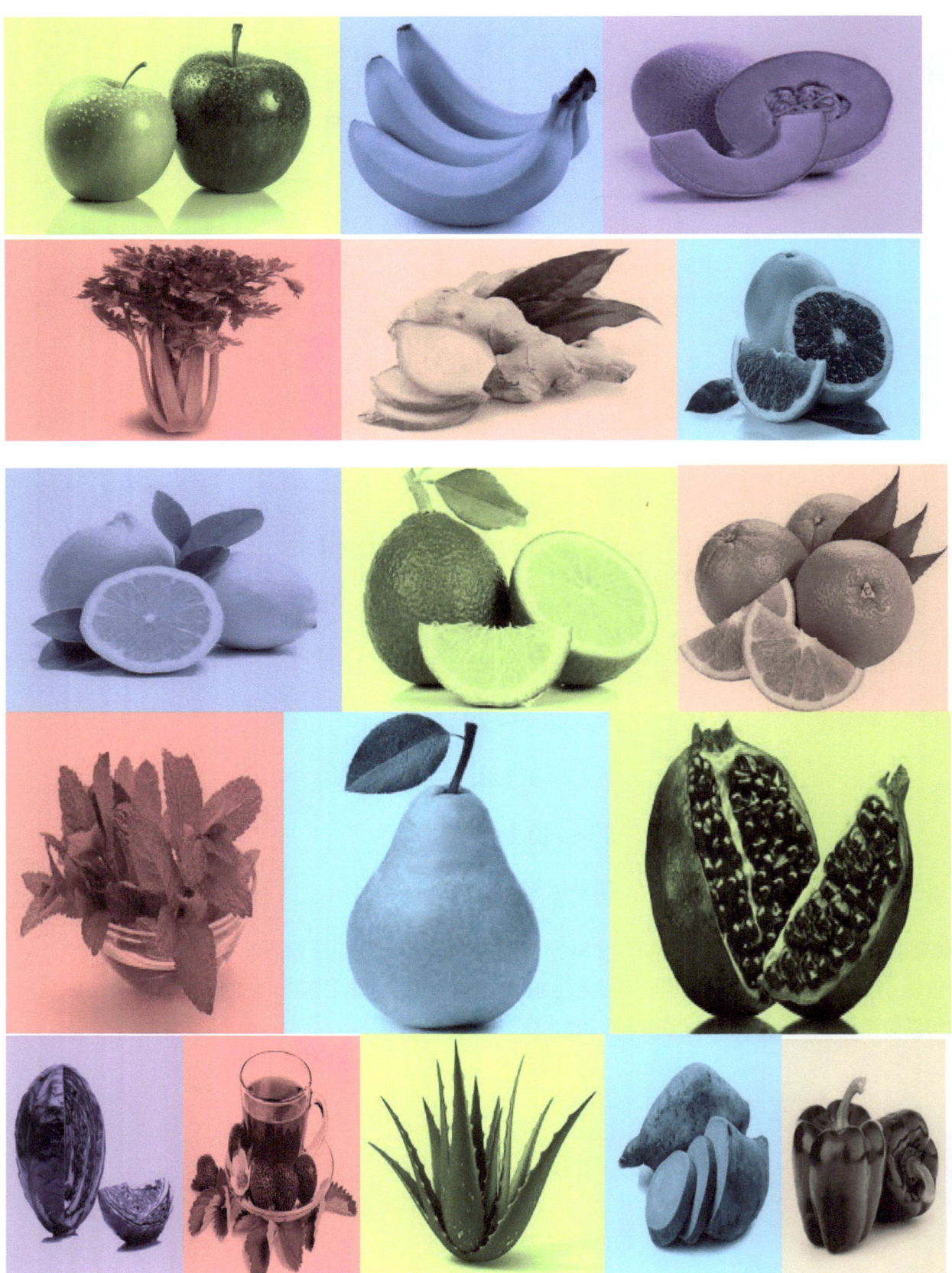

3

Nutritional Info

With everything new that you try always consult your physician first.

Sweet potatoes can be a good friend they are loaded with vitamin A and fiber.

Aloe Vera can be used as a daily vitamin loaded with vitamin A, C, and E amino acids and calcium.

Kale is high in Vitamin K and iron plus an excellent anti-inflammatory.

Beets are high in beta-carotene and magnesium. These fruits and vegetables are inexpensive and can be a preventive for many health issues. Enjoy your juicing and remember consult your physician.